HEAL
YOURSELF
ORACLE

T0405399

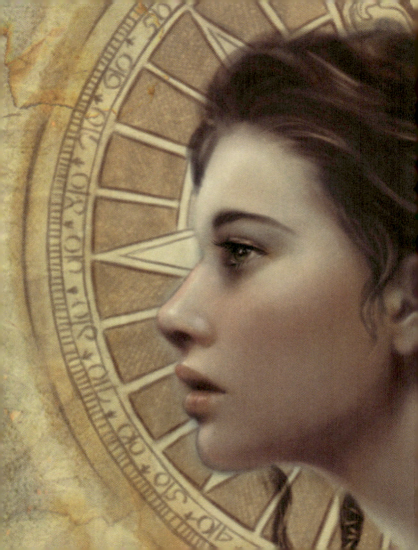

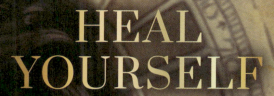

HEAL YOURSELF

ORACLE

**INTUITIVE GUIDANCE
TO TRANSFORM
YOUR SOUL**

INNA SEGAL

ROCKPOOL

To moving humanity forward!

INNA SEGAL

A Rockpool book
PO Box 252
Summer Hill NSW 2130
Australia

rockpoolpublishing.com
Follow us! f ⓘ rockpoolpublishing
Tag your images with #rockpoolpublishing

First published in 2017, by Rockpool Publishing, as Heal Yourself
Reading cards under ISBN 9781925017984

This edition published in 2024 by Rockpool Publishing

ISBN: 9781922785817

Copyright design © Rockpool Publishing 2024
Copyright text © Inna Segal 2017

Edited by Katie Evans
Design by Sara Lindberg, Rockpool Publishing

Artwork by Cris Ortega, crisortega.com,
pages 12, 14, 18, 20, 22, 24, 26, 28, 30, 32, 34, 36, 38, 40, 42, 44, 46, 50,
52, 54, 56, 62, 64, 66, 68, 70, 72, 74, 78, 80, 82

Artwork by Drazenka Kimpel, creativedust.com,
pages 16, 48, 58, 60, 76.

Printed and bound in China
10 9 8 7 6 5 4 3 2 1

CONTENTS

INTRODUCTION

My dear open-hearted reader, you are holding this booklet because there is a stirring deep inside your soul that says there is more to life than what you have experienced so far. You may not know exactly what you need to change, you may just feel that it is time for you to transform and to receive real self-love, intuitive guidance, courage and healing.

This deck is visceral, emotional and raw, expressing both the light and the darker sides of life. The cards empower you to access higher states of awareness as well as transform the challenging emotions, thought patterns and energies you are experiencing.

The cards give you insight into where you are in your life. They will magnify situations and show you the traits you may subconsciously be trying to disown. The purpose of each message is to bring you closer to your true self. I encourage you to take time to meditate on each card, its meaning and the image. If you experience a negative reaction to a card you have chosen, rather than rejecting it or thinking that it doesn't relate to you, stay with it, breathe and feel what it evokes.

Some of the themes I tackle are very delicate. In particular: how we sell out, our propensity to sabotage ourselves, our negative self-image and lack of self-love. I urge you to explore your sexuality, embrace your beauty, say what you mean and heal your childhood pain. Those are serious subjects, which require profound honesty on your part and a willingness to see the truth of your situation. The more you connect with and touch the deck, the more the cards will take on the role of your Higher Self, unveiling and amplifying the traits and aspects of your life you need to pay heed to. If a card brings up some deep feelings, I encourage you to find a therapist, a healer or a body worker to help you. You may also like to keep a journal, where you can record your journey of transformation.

As well as acknowledging your shadow aspects I encourage you to take charge of your life, be an artist and paint a new picture.

These cards differ from many other decks in that they require you to take genuine 'action' steps in order to transform. The steps are simple but profound.

I encourage you to take your time contemplating what the action step is asking you to do and repeat it several times until you feel that you have mastered it. You can combine the steps with other processes you know, in particular from my book *The Secret of Life Wellness* or *The Secret Language of Your Body*. These cards will only make a positive change in your life if you complete the processes.

If you love these cards and would like to explore deeper aspects of who you are please connect with me through my website www.innasegal.com. I have free videos as well as online seminars which tackle many of the subjects contained in this card deck.

I have based these cards on the different aspects of wellness, relationships, spirituality, love and soulfulness I have explored over many years. These themes have helped me transform many areas of my life, including excruciatingly painful health issues, disconnection from and hatred of my body, deteriorating relationships, abuse, sexual shame, rejection of my femininity, childhood trauma and many other powerful experiences. Some themes I have explored for many months, others for years, many I continue to work on.

The cards remind us of the truth, which is stored in our bodies. This truth will set us free when we are willing to offer it the same attention and energy we give the falsehoods that keep us small. No one can make you change, only you can choose to open your heart and mind towards real transformation and become whole.

HOW TO USE THE CARDS

One card reading

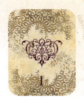

This card deck can be used daily. Ask a question, mentally, shuffle the cards then pull out a card you feel drawn to. Focus on the picture on the card and meditate on how it makes you feel and how the message relates to you. Then read the guidebook and complete the exercise associated with the card.

The exercises are very powerful and can transform your life so make sure you take the time to do them properly. You can complete the exercise once on the day you pick the card or you may decide to repeat it every day that week.

Three or four card reading

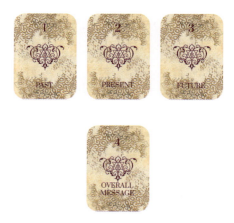

Choose three cards – one to represent the past, one to represent the present and one to represent the future.

The card on the left will show you the origin of the situation (past), the middle card will describe where you are at and what you need to focus on presently (present), the card on the right will show possibilities of a future outcome (future). If you feel guided you can also pick a fourth card that will show you the overall message you need to understand.

If a card you pick is upside down then it will show you that this is an area where you are being challenged and that you really need to work with the process described regularly and make life changes. I would suggest to work with the process between 7 and 30 days.

PENDULUM

Spread the cards in a circle and hold a pendulum over the cards (such as a locket on a chain). Ask a question and notice which card the pendulum swings towards.

JUMPING CARD

If when shuffling a card jumps out of the deck it usually means you need to pay attention to the message on that particular card.

REPEATED MESSAGE

If you repeatedly choose the same card then you need to read it carefully two or three times, engage deeply with the process prescribed for the card and reflect on what it is telling you.

ENERGY READING

If you are someone who feels energy, lay out the cards and move your hands, palms down, just above them. Once you feel a tingling sensation or some warmth, choose the card where the sensation was felt. When you pick it up, look at the picture and become conscious of the message the picture is giving you. Be aware of your feelings and sensations. Then read the meaning. You can pick one card or several.

FUTURE READING

For future readings clarify if you would like a message that is related to a month, six months, a year or longer from now.

CHOICE

This is a six-card spread. Decide on a problem or issue and think of two outcomes or choices that are possible.

Focus on choice one and pick three cards and place them on top of the deck, facing up.

Card 1 will show you what is possible in relation to choice one.

Card 2 will show you what lessons you will need to learn or challenges you will need to overcome in relation to choice one.

Card 3 will show you the possible outcome of this choice.

Reshuffle the cards. Focus on choice two and pick three new cards and place them on top of the deck, facing up.

Card 1 will show you what is possible in relation to choice two.

Card 2 will show you what lessons you will need to learn or challenges you will need to overcome in relation to choice two.

Card 3 will show you the possible outcome of this choice.

If you already know of any other ways to read your cards, feel free to apply those reading formats to this deck. The intention of the deck is to create positive change in your life.

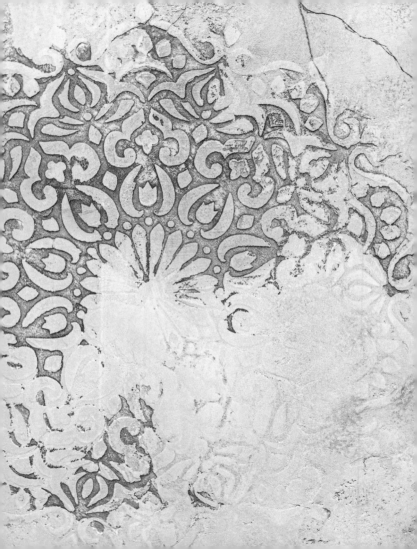

HEAL YOURSELF

ORACLE CARDS

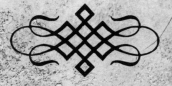

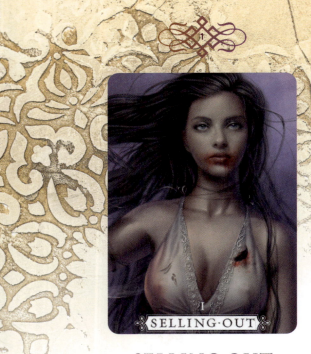

SELLING OUT

Your integrity and inner strength are being severely tested.
You have an opportunity to act with either fear or love.

Where in your life are you selling out or acting out of integrity? Are you in a job you hate? Are you living in a toxic environment and making yourself sick in the pursuit of financial security?

This card asks you to find the courage to stand up for your convictions and take steps towards doing what you love.

Selling out is linked to the shadow aspect of the Prostitute archetype. When you connect to this archetype you can examine your fears around survival, power, responsibility and success.

On the light side, the Prostitute can lead you to freedom, self-expression, choice and love.

ACTION

You have to make a choice about whether you will use your power, talents and abilities for selfishness and exploitation or the higher good?

Take a few deep breaths and focus on your body. Become conscious of where in your body you feel like you are losing your energy and your power.

Place your hands on that part of your body.

Visualise your Prostitute archetype; it can look similar to this card or a darker version of you. Ask this archetype to show you where in your life you are selling out. Become aware of how this affects various areas of your life and your physical and emotional health.

Ask your Prostitute aspect to help you regain your inner strength and make empowering decisions.

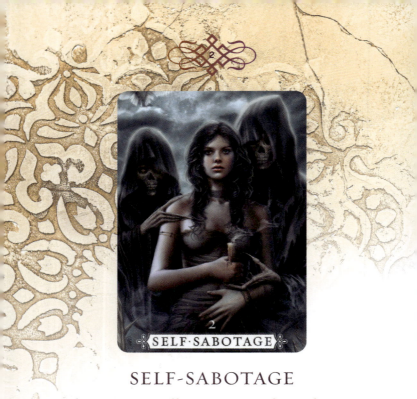

SELF-SABOTAGE

Become conscious of how your inner saboteur functions.
You are about to sabotage a big opportunity.

Now is the time to stop procrastinating and cease focusing your energy on why you are unworthy of wonderful, enriching experiences.

When you connect to the Saboteur archetype you begin to recognise all the ways you pass up interesting opportunities and relationships which could make you grow, learn, evolve and become fulfilled.

The Saboteur is terrified of change and guards your heart from that which is meaningful to you, with the misguided belief that if you don't try you can't fail. It forgets that if you don't escape from your comfort zone you cannot succeed and experience the love and joy, which would fulfil you.

On the lighter side the Saboteur can help you connect to your intuition and help you to listen to your deeper wisdom. It can assist you in deciphering a potentially dangerous situation from an exciting one.

ACTION

Take a few deep breaths and become conscious of where in your body you feel like you are limiting yourself.

Place your hands on that part of your body.

Visualise your Saboteur archetype; it may look similar to this card or like a shadow aspect of you. Ask this part of yourself to show you how you miss out on or sabotage your relationships, career, money, health and any other aspects of your life where you are not fulfilled. Become aware of your patterns. Make a commitment to yourself to start focusing on your strengths rather than your weaknesses and welcome new experiences into your life.

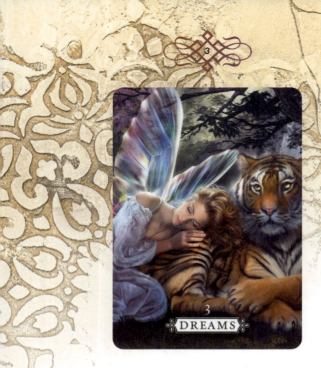

DREAMS

Pay attention to your dreams – they hold lots of significant insights for you at present.

Your dreams may provide you with important details about your current health issues or a creative idea you need to action to make your desires manifest. Dreams can also give you clues about what is challenging you emotionally.

Sometimes your loved ones who have passed over or people you have lost touch with connect to you while you sleep and offer valuable messages that can give you peace of mind or the strength to persist through a challenging situation.

Take note of both the dark and the light aspects of your dreams. In particular, pay attention to any recurring dreams as they often have significant meaning or wisdom that can help you.

ACTION

Before going to sleep place a glass of water next to your bed, position this card over the water with an intention to remember your dreams. Let the card energise the water. Then take a few sips of the water.

Relax and think about a question you would like answered.

You can write your question in a notebook, or repeat the question to yourself as you drift off to sleep.

In the morning, drink some water from the glass and write down anything you can remember from your dreams.

Be particularly aware of the feelings associated with a specific scene in your dream. It can reveal a great deal about how you unconsciously feel about yourself and the people in your life.

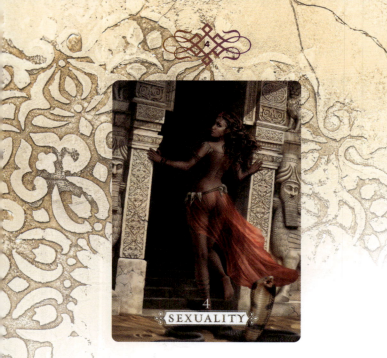

SEXUALITY

Sexuality is a natural part of life. Embrace and enjoy your intimate, sensual, passionate nature.

Take time to explore your sexuality. How do you feel about yourself? Do you feel sexy, attractive and happy with your body, or are you judging yourself harshly?

You need to let go of any old feelings of hurt, shame or guilt in relation to your sexuality.

If you are in a relationship you need to bring some romance back and spice things up. In order to make sex an incredibly fulfilling, seductive, exhilarating and orgasmic experience you need to let go of your defences and fears of being intimate with your partner. Relinquish control and dive into unguarded, ecstatic, blissful passion. Be creative, communicate with your lover and find new and exciting ways to thrill each other.

ACTION

You need to love your body. Stand in front of the mirror, naked, and discover what is beautiful about your physical appearance. Place your hands on your sacral centre, put on some sexy music and move in a sensual, creative, uninhibited way. Do this every day for the next two weeks.

If you are in a relationship make a romantic date with your partner that will include some love and passion. Start with a sensual or an erotic massage and take it further. Ask each other what will give you pleasure and be willing to be creative and try new things! If you are game, explore the power of feminine and masculine polarities!

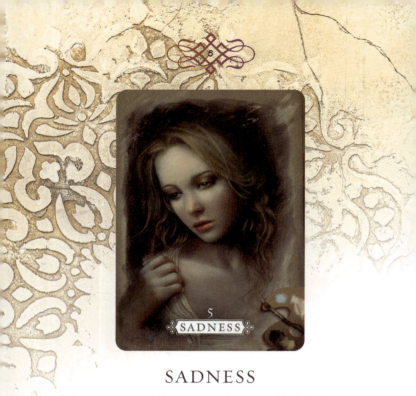

SADNESS

*It's easy to swallow your sadness and hide behind
a fake smile. Yet sadness can open the door to
your heart and help you access compassion.*

When you can truly allow yourself to cry and feel sorrow over the loss of a loved one, a lost opportunity, a broken heart or a friendship that's ended, you cleanse your soul and allow your heart to heal.

Crying and feeling vulnerable can be a sign of strength which demonstrates your connection to your body.

To admit weakness can allow you to know yourself, embrace your limitations and evolve.

Be willing to let go of the cold walls of protection you have created, which make you feel empty and sick.

You don't need to get lost in your emotions, just give yourself time to feel them and let them move through your whole being, cleansing and purifying your heart, body and soul.

ACTION

Relax your body. Place your hands on your heart. Ask yourself, 'Where am I holding on to feelings of loss, grief and sadness?' Have you frozen your tears and cut yourself off from your feelings because you are afraid to face a person or a situation?

Put on some music or a song that touches you and imagine taking off the layers of protection from your heart. Then rub your hands together for 30 seconds, place your hands next to each other palms inwards and imagine holding a bright yellow ball of light in between your palms. Place your hands on your heart and allow this yellow light to dissolve any iciness from your heart.

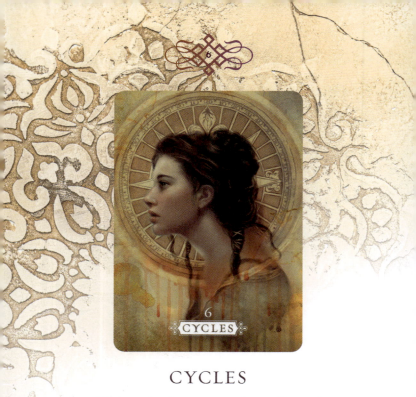

CYCLES

*Life is cyclical, sometimes things flow and
at other times they slow down.*

What cycle of your life are you in right now? What is the one area of
your life where you need to focus most of your energy?

Is it time for you to focus on your family? Do you need alone time to discover your true purpose? Do you yearn to open your heart and love fully, deeply and passionately? Is this the time for healing and regeneration?

Maybe you are completely ready to enthusiastically concentrate on your life purpose and put all your energy and effort into making your dreams a reality.

Each cycle you encounter offers you fresh gifts and possibilities to learn and grow. The better you become at identifying the cycle you are in, the more flow and harmony you will experience in the choices you make.

ACTION

Your body is the key to showing you where you are at. Do you have the energy and the vitality to focus on your goals or are you in a period of healing?

Write down what you are experiencing at present. Read over what you wrote several times. Then give yourself permission to honour the cycle you are in. Is it time to learn or to apply what you have learned?

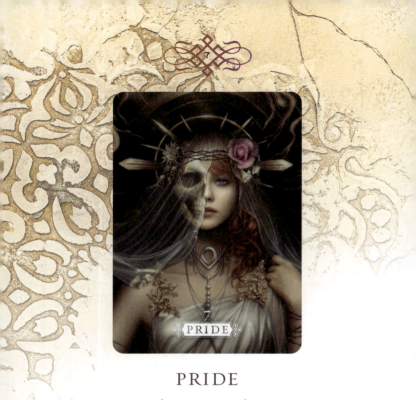

PRIDE

*You may be acting out of arrogance
and vanity. Humility is the key.*

When you are prideful you can become harsh and not conscious of
your weaknesses. This can temporarily make you feel more powerful

and superior to others, whilst at the same time cause you to be judgemental, unteachable and hardened.

Have you been fighting, quarrelling and disagreeing with others? Are you always trying to prove a point and defend your position? Do you think that you are always right?

By holding on to shadow pride you are stopping yourself from progressing mentally, emotionally and spiritually.

Stop overestimating your importance and learn to be humble. When you are too proud you cannot hear other people's advice and cannot receive their assistance. Empowerment means that you can be soft, caring, aware and gentle. Recognise that you need other people's support to achieve true success.

ACTION

Take some time during the day to relax. Lie down if possible and look carefully at this card. How does it make you feel? How do you relate to it?

Ask yourself, 'Where am I attached to a false sense of who I am? Where have I overestimated my abilities or charged ahead unprepared for the challenges I face? Where in the past has a sense of pride led me to a fall?'

Instead of taking this personally, now is your opportunity to feel and express your willingness to release any pride that has held you back and in doing so become more teachable. If you have hurt other people consider apologising and being more thoughtful.

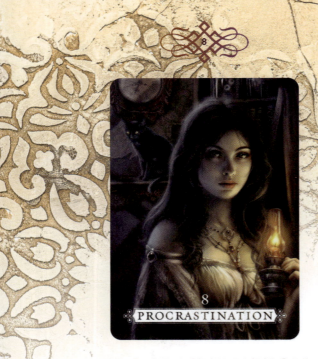

PROCRASTINATION

*You need to change your tune and stop putting
things off to tomorrow that you can do today.*

You are being called to action. There have been important tasks that
you have delayed.

Even if it is something that you don't want to do, like cleaning the house, paying the bills, looking for a job, losing weight, doing your tax, studying and so on, now is the time to take responsibility and move forward.

The point of power is always in the present. This card is showing you that there is an urgency for you to take action.

If you are putting off something that is meaningful to you and doubting whether you can do it, the message is to have courage to face your fears and do what you love. What is the worst thing that can happen? You make a mistake. Even if you do, you will learn.

ACTION

Make a list of all the tasks you have put off. Make another list of the things you have started and have not completed, then write a third list of things you would love to do.

Then write down what actions you can take today to free your mind and shorten that list. Which actions will you take in the next week?

Make a grounded, practical plan and for the next week or two keep this card close to you and look at it every time you become lazy and delay things you have to do.

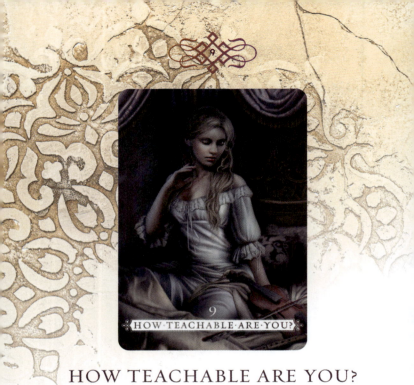

HOW TEACHABLE ARE YOU?

Are you open to learning new things in your life?
How high is your desire to let go of judgement,
doubt, negativity and self-sabotage?

What are some of your favourite things to do? Is it to watch TV, go shopping, play golf, drink, gossip with your friends? Are you willing to give those things up in order to create time to learn something new?

Are you sick and tired of being sick and tired? What is your willingness to really apply what you learn?

You might be learning many new things but are resistant to change. Every time you begin to think 'I already know this, I've heard it before, this doesn't apply to me', your ability to learn diminishes enormously and it is at this point you may become virtually unteachable without realising it. Unless you apply what you have learnt into your life, you won't really know it.

This card is beckoning you to not only be open-minded but to take specific action towards change.

ACTION

To create change you need to start with something small and eventually you will change your habit. This builds confidence as you start working towards the big changes you need to make.

In the next 48 hours take a step forward towards changing some area of your life. This could be something small like buying a journal to write your dreams in, or talking to someone about your transformation.

Then every day do something towards creating positive transformation in your life.

Another thing you can do is ask yourself many times during the day, 'Am I teachable right now?' People who are the most teachable experience the most success in their life!

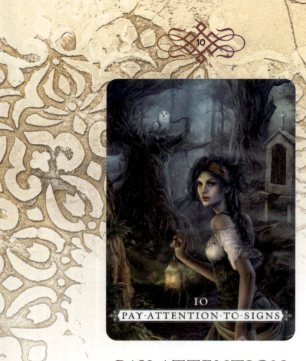

10

PAY·ATTENTION·TO·SIGNS

PAY ATTENTION
TO SIGNS

*Signs are all around you. Open your mind and
pay closer attention to your environment.*

Your angels know that you have been feeling lost about the direction
you need to take in your life and the decisions you need to make.

They have heard your frustrations and your pleas for help. They ask you to slow down, stop focusing on the problem and allow a solution to come into your reality.

Your spiritual helpers have been organising synchronistic events and support for you, but you keep thinking in the same stubborn way. Relax and look at life in a more creative way.

Pay attention to repetitive signs and signals. A sign can come in the form of a song, a movie, a book, nature, animals, people, thoughts, dreams, visions and so on.

At times your body also gives you signs. Your body may be telling you to rest, change your diet or to work on challenging emotions. Be sure to take these signals seriously.

ACTION

Do this with a friend: Put on a song. Dance freely. Have your friend stop the song between 2-3 minutes. When the music stops, make a gesture. From that position think about your challenge from a different perspective. Ask for a sign then repeat the exercise with a new song 4-5 times. Record all important insights.

Over the next week pay attention to signs from your environment as well as from your dreams.

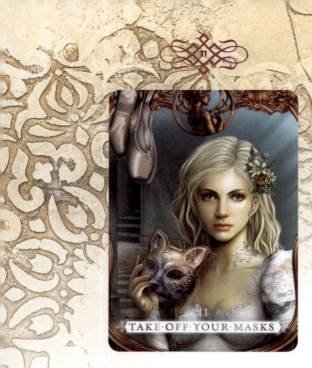

TAKE OFF YOUR MASK(S)

Stop trying to appear different to who you really are.
It's time to take off your mask and be the real you.

You cannot get the love and attention you are craving by pretending to be someone you are not.

Why are you so frightened to be honest with yourself and others? Do you feel that you will lose friends and opportunities by showing others your imperfections, fears and vulnerabilities?

Are you constantly doing things to please others even if doing this does not work for you?

This card indicates that you need time to get to know yourself and what is important in your life.

You will know that you are evolving when other people's judgements of you no longer impact you.

If you have an incredible talent, believe in yourself! Don't hide your greatness because others feel envious or resentful. Remember, every great leader had people who loved them and believed in them as well as those who doubted and disliked them.

ACTION

Take a few deep breaths and focus on your body. Reflect upon in which areas of your life you are wearing masks and not being authentic.

Think of different situations that make you feel vulnerable. Imagine taking off the masks that you wear and speaking honestly with kindness to a particular person who intimidates you. Take back your power.

Give yourself permission to be real and to say what you mean, from a place of gentleness and compassion.

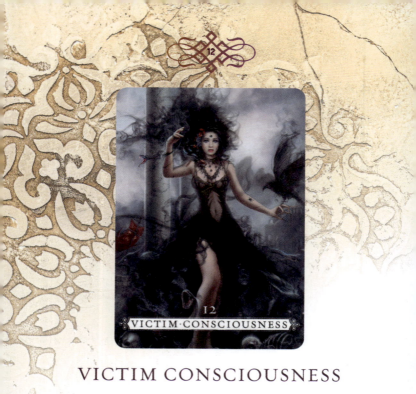

VICTIM CONSCIOUSNESS

*Stop blaming others and take responsibility
for what you are creating.*

It's easy to think that life is unfair and point a finger at others. If
you hear yourself saying, 'Life is unfair. Bad things always happen to
me. I'm not good enough, nobody cares about me. Why me? I can't

do what I want to do' and so on then you are losing your power, nourishing your victim aspect and ascertaining your place in the victim club.

Your inner victim can stop you from moving forward by creating dramas, making you judge others, telling you that you don't deserve better and keeping you stuck in a financial rut.

You need to build your internal confidence, self-worth and courage. Get out of your comfort zone and work on expanding and growing in all areas of your life.

The light side of the Victim archetype is the victorious part, which can help you to hold your power without getting angry and attacking others. It can also assist you to create healthy boundaries and act from a place of honesty, integrity, compassion and love.

ACTION

Visualise your inner victim. Ask to be aware when you are acting like a victim. Then ask your inner victim to show you how you could behave in a more empowered way. How do you need to think, feel and act to be empowered?

On a daily basis ask yourself, 'Am I acting from an empowered, victorious perspective or a victim perspective?'

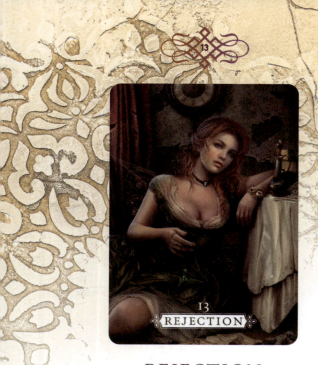

REJECTION

Use rejection to grow, expand and build yourself.

Feeling rejected can disconnect you from your heart and soul and immobilise you.

Rather than buying into rejection, focus on how you can grow, learn and improve from your experiences. If you are a writer and you sent your articles or a book to a publisher and they have rejected it, then try to hone your writing skills and then send your work out to several other publishers. Use that rejection as a motivating force to succeed.

If a person that you have feelings for or felt a deep love towards has rejected you, then work on healing your heart and recognising that there is someone out there who is more suited to you.

Many people use rejection as an excuse to close down, become suspicious, guarded and give up. Then they hurt and reject others. They hide behind rejection and never give themselves an opportunity to take a leap of faith and find their life calling and heal.

By picking this card you are being urged to hold yourself in a higher regard. Keep your heart open and trust that you have learnt from your experiences and will not make the same mistakes again.

ACTION

Take a pen and paper. On one side of the paper write down what you are afraid of, especially in terms of being rejected. On the other side record how you can use rejection to succeed then take action with confidence that rejection can be your friend.

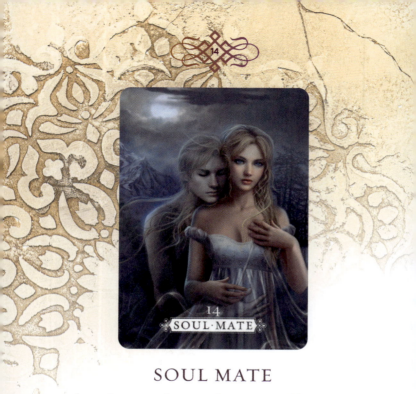

SOUL MATE

Open your heart and invite sacred love.

Your soul mate is not far from you. To connect with them you need to open your heart, call them in and have patience. If you are not ready to accept your soul mate, keep working on self-love.

You will be drawn to your soul mate like a magnet and feel an immense sense of familiarity, like you have known them before. Your capacity to love will increase dramatically and you will experience higher states of consciousness. No one can touch your heart in the same way that a soul mate can.

It is important to note that your soul mate will not necessarily be your partner. He or she may come in a completely different form than you have imagined, but they will offer you incredible wisdom, growth and expansion.

Be aware that we connect with our soul mates when we are ready to truly evolve and move to the next level of consciousness and life experience. We attract them into our lives when we need to open our hearts fully and learn about unconditional love.

ACTION

Take some slow deep breaths. Connect to your heart. Imagine calling your soul mate towards you. You don't have to know what they look like, just feel the openness in your heart and allow yourself to connect to their heart. Imagine that there is a gold cord attaching you to them, with beautiful loving energy flowing between you.

Know that you are supported and will soon meet each other in the physical reality.

Keep working on opening your heart and enjoying your life.

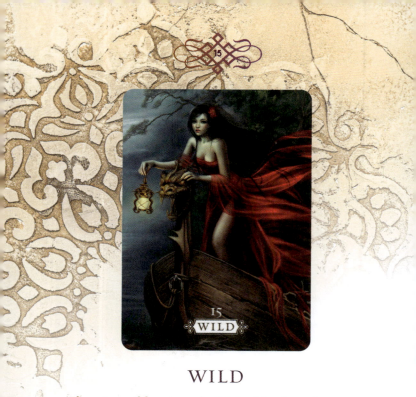

WILD

There is a wild, untamed spirit inside of you desperate to be unleashed. Free it and claim the gifts of energy, power, passion and creativity it offers you.

Through suppressing your wild, succulent, outrageous and untamed self, you dull your senses and crush your creativity. You shrink, lose your energy and become depressed. Your relationships suffer and your rage grows. You become ashamed, hostile, cold, boring, over serious and scared. You stop taking chances and live in mediocrity, constantly trying to protect yourself. The truth is that no one can judge you, punish you or hurt you as much as you can.

Give in to your wildness and stop living a sham. This part of you is sensual, provocative, truthful, courageous, bold, passionate and alive. Set it free!

ACTION

Go into nature – a forest is ideal. Find a secluded place. Take off your shoes. Feel the earth or the grass underneath your feet. Breathe in the air.

Connect to the untamed quality of nature, animals, weather, seasons, planets and your ancestors. Move the way tribal people move. Feel the energy from the ground moving into your feet and up your whole body. Make sounds. Let go of control as you move around, touching trees, smelling flowers and so on.

If you want to do this inside, find photos of people, animals or symbols which represent wildness to you. Take a few minutes to look at them and feel what they evoke in you. Put on some tribal or wild music and dance. Do this as often as you can for the next month.

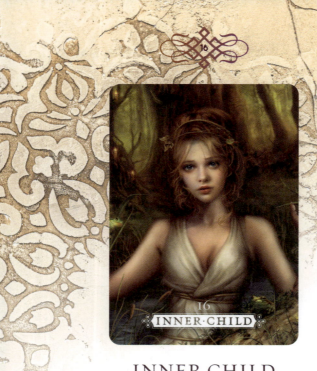

INNER CHILD

*Your inner child is urging you to lighten up a little,
get out of your comfort zone and have fun!*

In order to be healthy we must engage our imagination, creativity
and spontaneity.

When was the last time you did something spontaneous, intuitive and outrageous?

When and with whom do you feel uninhibited, relaxed and completely comfortable to be yourself?

Your inner child can be your strongest ally or your biggest foe. It can assist you to heal childhood pain, rejection, loneliness and abandonment. It can take you on an exciting adventure, help you become more confident, daring, original and bold. Or it can make you behave in childish ways; bring up anxiety, fear and suspicion.

This card beckons you to heal your childhood pain and discover your independence, compassion, creativity, talents and joy. A healthy inner child can help you connect to your integrity, Divinity and purity. It believes in miracles and creates magic in your life.

ACTION

Find a photo of you as a child between the ages of three and eight. Look at the picture. What do you see in your eyes? What is the expression on your face? If this little child had a voice what would she/he say to you? Take some paper and, using your non-dominant hand, write: Dear _____ (your name) I feel … Give the 'little' you a chance to express itself. Then write a loving response from the adult you.

Ask the child in you what she/he needs to feel better. Then follow the child's recommendation.

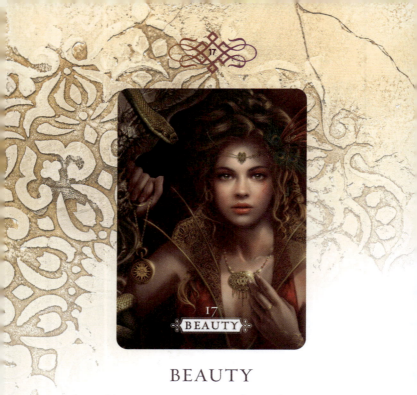

BEAUTY

Recognise your inner and outer beauty.

You are beautiful, special, unique and attractive.

When was the last time you looked in the mirror and felt good about what you see? Did you know that your features can literally change based on how you feel about yourself and your life?

Your internal experiences are etched on your face and your body. People can feel your energy when you enter a room. When a person who is not thought of as being physically good looking connects to their own inner light, wisdom and warmth, the glow that emanates from within makes them extremely appealing and attracts people and opportunities towards them.

Focus on what you love about yourself and allow yourself to shine. If you are challenged by how you see yourself this could be a perfect time for an internal and an external makeover.

ACTION

Look at your face in the mirror. Acknowledge what is beautiful about you. It can be physical or spiritual.

Ask yourself how you nurture your internal beauty. Do you allow others to see your light, your caring side, kindness and warmth?

Ask your body what it needs to feel healthy and taken care of. This could involve changing your diet, having a new exercise program, updating your wardrobe, getting a new haircut and so on.

Give to yourself.

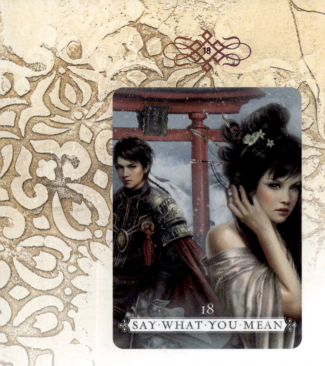

SAY WHAT YOU MEAN

*Take some time to clarify what you need
to communicate and to whom.*

Honest communication begins with you. Take a moment to connect
within and ask yourself, in what area of your life are you hiding and

denying how you feel? Does your relationship with your partner need revamping? Are there things that are not working?

Who are the people in your life that you must be honest with? This is your opportunity to take back your power and share clearly, wisely and honestly what does and does not work for you.

When you feel vulnerable you can be easily swayed to say what you feel the other person wants to hear in order to keep the peace. The message of this card is that you need to say what you really mean whether someone else likes it or not.

ACTION

Rub your hands together for about 30-40 seconds then imagine that you are holding a blue ball of energy in your hands. Reflect on the qualities of confidence, honesty and clarity. Then place your hands just above your throat and breathe in the blue light. Imagine this light moving into your throat and helping you to access the right words that you need to say.

Picture the person who you need to communicate with standing in front of you. Share what you feel you need to say to this person, realising that their Higher Self is listening.

When you have completed this action, write down what you feel you need to say to them. Then share your feelings in person if appropriate.

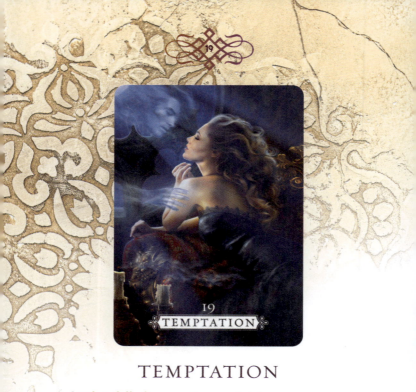

TEMPTATION

*Life is full of temptations and right now you are
being asked to choose the higher path.*

Your need to prove that you are worthy and important is clouding
your true purpose and tempting you to make wrong decisions.

Become aware of what is happening in your life right now. Are you feeling bored in a relationship and looking for something outside of your partnership instead of being honest and working on the challenges you are experiencing, or moving on?

Is there a work opportunity that is tempting you to act without integrity in order to get ahead?

Are you using money as an excuse not to follow your heart?

This card asks you to focus on the bigger picture, be honest with yourself and take the higher path.

Another opportunity that is much grander than what you have imagined is on its way, just be open to it and allow it into your life.

ACTION

Give yourself 5 minutes of uninterrupted time. Write down in what area of your life you are being tempted, what choices you have made and what are the best choices you could make.

Rub your hands together then place them slightly apart from each other. Imagine that you are holding an orange ray of light between your hands. Focus on courage. What does it mean for you to be courageous enough not to buy into temptation? Place your hands on the part of your body where you need courage the most. Send the orange ray there and repeat, 'I am courageous and take positive actions that yield the greatest results.' Imagine yourself acting courageously and doing what will lead you to the higher path.

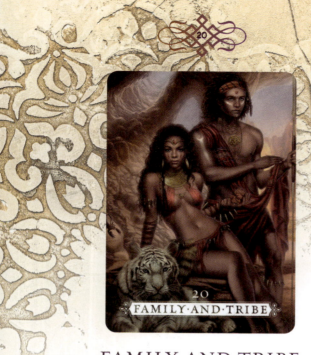

FAMILY AND TRIBE

Be very discerning with other people's opinions.

Become aware of how the beliefs of your family and tribe are influencing you. What did you learn about relationships, money and opportunities when you were younger?

Ask yourself, 'Am I still carrying some of those outdated beliefs? Am I trying to seek love and approval from my family by doing what they want me to do?'

An important question to ask yourself is whether you are living your life in order to make someone else or yourself happy.

This card asks you to examine your loyalties, family beliefs, superstitions and rituals that have power over you. Let go of anything that is not serving you. You are also being asked to face your fears of being different and embrace your uniqueness even if others don't understand or approve of your actions.

Working often with your energy centres, in particular the root chakra, can help you release past limitations and hurts, increase your confidence and help you manifest your desires into the physical reality.

ACTION

Recognise beliefs that you have adopted from others. Play some tribal music. Imagine that other people's limiting beliefs are like chains that stop you from moving forward. Stamp your feet and focus on recognising each belief, pattern or past experience and then imagine letting them go. You can even visualise throwing all the chains into a purple flame which dissolves them.

Then give yourself permission to move forward and put all of your energy, on a daily basis, into how you would love to live your life.

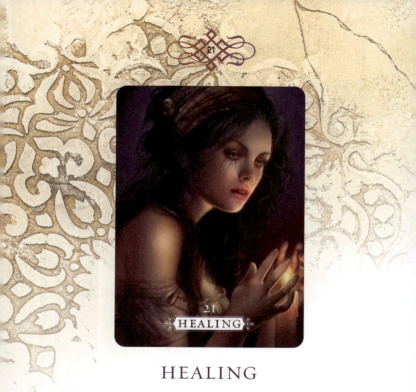

HEALING

Illness and pain in your body is a message for you to slow down, look within and make important changes.

If you are experiencing stress, feel overwhelmed, are suffering ailments in your body, or feel exhausted and depressed, it means that your body is trying to communicate with you.

Your body wants you to start treating it in a more loving manner and listening to the messages it is sending you. You need to become conscious of the areas in your life that you are avoiding or suppressing.

Healing takes time. It is a process. Your first step towards healing is to create a safe, loving, supportive environment, where you can listen to your inner wisdom.

ACTION

Take a few deep breaths and relax your body. Place your hands on an area in your body where you have pain.

Ask your body, 'Is there a message you want to give me?' This message may come to you as thoughts, words, images, insights, feelings, memories and so on.

Say, 'I call on my Divine Healing Intelligence to help release all pain, blockages and density from this area.' Watch and feel as dense energy leaves your body.

Say, 'I call on my Divine Healing Intelligence to infuse this area with a green ray of light. I ask that all the immune mechanisms of my body be activated and my body now returns to a state of perfect balance and health.'

Imagine a green light moving through your body and repairing it. Gently bring your awareness back to normal and open your eyes.

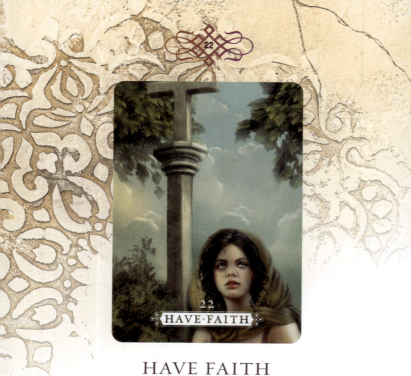

HAVE FAITH

*Faith requires you to believe in something
that is not yet evident to the naked eye.*

To generate more faith focus on the WHY: your dreams, desires,
feelings, attitudes and thinking, and not on the HOW: action plan,
strategies and skills. Your whole life you have been taught to think

about the 'how', which leads to doubt and fear. The wisdom of this card is asking you to only focus on the 'why'!

The magic that will happen if you stop focusing on the 'how' and only on the 'why' is that after some time of practice you will notice that the 'how' will present itself to you.

It is through your focused, positive thinking that you will create people, circumstances and events that will take you closer to your dreams. What you have mostly done is to focus on the 'how', which has made you doubt yourself. This means that you are vibrating negative thoughts into the universe, keeping your dreams away. Remember you were created to be a co-creator here on earth, designed for achievement. Faith is knowing that everything is going to work out the best possible way no matter what things look like.

ACTION

Take a sheet of paper and in seven minutes write down (not on a computer) all the things you would do or be or have if money and time were not obstacles. Do this exercise every day for one week. Then, at the end of each entry, write a number between 1 and 10 (10 being you definitely could make this happen within six months, and 1 being there is no chance you could achieve this goal in six months). Pick entries that are marked 7 or above and find one to focus your energy on. Soon the 'how' will present itself and you will take a huge step closer to your most treasured dreams. This will build massive confidence and increased faith in the magic of the universe.

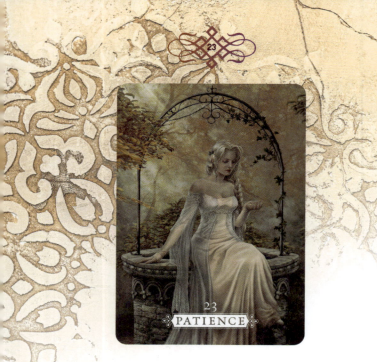

PATIENCE

You must develop patience in all areas of your life.

Patience does not mean that you give up and do nothing. On the contrary, you need to be aware of several aspects of the circumstance that you are facing. Patience requires you to stop pushing, rushing and creating potentially explosive situations. Instead it asks you to see the bigger picture and become aware of the ingredients that might be missing.

If you are impatient with a particular person, instead give them space.

Avoid jumping to conclusions and making up dramatic stories about a person or a situation without being aware of all the details. You have an opportunity to let go of judgement. Always look for the truth of the situation, not what someone is saying or doing, but why?

Patience can also be connected to a health condition you are recovering from, a new diet or an exercise program you have embarked on, or a new course of study you may have begun.

ACTION

Focus on one thing at a time.

Say to yourself, 'I accept what is without judgement. I am willing to practise patience and presence.'

Breathe slowly and deeply while focusing on what is. Be aware of the air hitting your nostrils and lungs. Soften and relax. Be the explorer of the present moment. Discover what is magical, beautiful and serene in this moment. If you are feeling unwell or stressed, just allow yourself to explore these feelings with the awareness that they will pass.

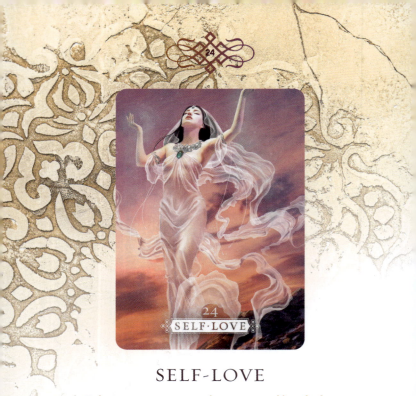

SELF-LOVE

Take time out to get to know yourself and what
works for you in this particular cycle of your life.

Some of the biggest obstacles to self-love are self-criticism and
perfectionism, which lead to harsh judgement of the self, closing
down, and, eventually, illness. Have you been trying to compete with

others, get approval from people in your family or simply pushing yourself too hard? If so, you need to soften and start listening to your body. Focus on keeping your heart open and practise acknowledging and recognising the good in yourself and others.

This card beckons you to breathe love in and out every moment of the day. Ask yourself, 'What changes do I need to make to my daily routine so that love can pulsate through every breath, action and relationship I engage in?'

Choose to open your heart through softness, deep breathing, relaxation, movement, finding beauty in nature, in your home, in your pain, in your love, in your sadness, in prayer and so on. Keep your heart open even though it makes you feel vulnerable and exposed.

ACTION

This week is your opportunity to learn to receive. Any time anyone says something nice to you or offers to help you, take a deep breath, thank them and accept. You need to find something loving or nurturing to do for yourself. This could be a massage, a healing treatment or a movie with a friend.

Every time you look in the mirror, repeat, 'I am lovable.' Do this every day until you really believe it.

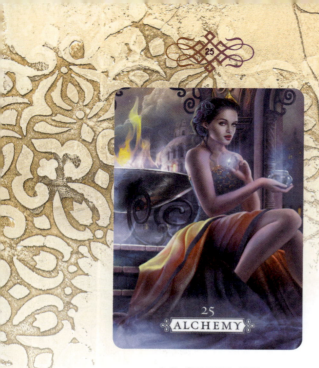

ALCHEMY

The path you are on is about to go through a very powerful transformation. Nothing is how it seems.

You have an opportunity to take a big leap in your level of consciousness. It is extremely important that you focus on letting go of any negativity and beliefs that no longer serve you.

You have access to the energy of alchemy, which can transform the most challenging experiences into incredible gifts and miracles.

Meditate and take action on your highest goals and dreams. They are on their way to coming true.

Let go of your expectations. What is about to appear can surpass anything you have dreamed of. The most important part is that you are prepared, and ready to receive.

The energy around you is very potent at the moment so make sure that you are using this time as productively as possible.

Give yourself time for prayer, gratitude and celebration.

ACTION

Rub your hands together vigorously for 40 seconds, then place your hands a few centimetres apart. Visualise a golden ball of light. Focus your intention on what you would like to create and place this intention into the golden light. Then move your hands towards your heart. Feel your heart expand and grow full. Ask your Higher Self to guide you towards your deepest expansion and evolution.

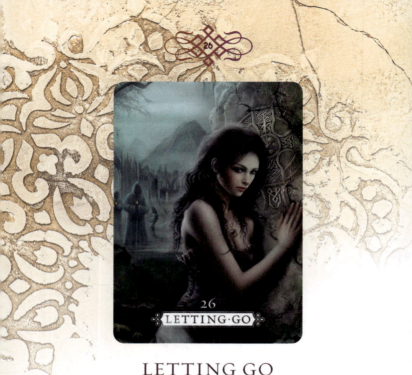

LETTING GO

This situation has served its purpose.

You are being challenged to change your point of view and recognise that this particular relationship has run its course. Although you might be afraid to let go, the universe has a new opportunity for you, which will allow you to experience the kind of passion and satisfaction you have always dreamed of.

Saying goodbye is never easy and can make you feel like you are a failure. You must not allow yourself to be persuaded by other people or your own doubts, to keep holding on.

Focus on opening your heart to a new opportunity. Leave the baggage of past mistakes behind you.

It is important that during the 'letting go' process you are gentle with yourself. Allow yourself to have alone time – write, meditate, paint, sing, dance. Do whatever you can to heal and let go of the pain that is holding you back. Recognise that your spirit is beckoning you to grow.

ACTION

When you feel stuck in a point of view, you can ask yourself, 'Is this my belief or someone else's? How does it serve me? Am I willing to let go of my fears and unfounded limitations?'

Say, 'Divine Healing Intelligence please assist me to let go of this situation_____(state what it is), habit (state what it is) _____, person (say their name)_____ with ease and grace. Inspire me to move forward with freedom, lightness and a feeling of completion. Bring into my reality new and empowering experiences, people and opportunities. Thank you.' Repeat the word 'clear' several times.

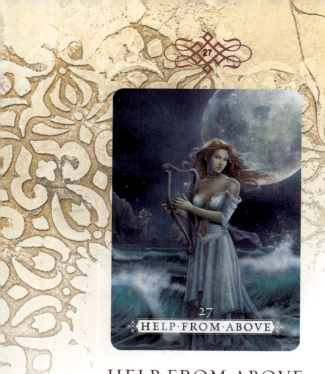

HELP FROM ABOVE

*Your positive intentions and heartfelt
prayers have been heard.*

You are loved beyond your wildest dreams. Divine beings are working
on your behalf to create the perfect circumstances for you to heal and
open your heart. There is a Higher Order and timing to all things.

You are being asked to work on your self-worth, so that you can receive your greatest good in the form of incredible love, life transforming opportunities, healing, abundance and Divine inspiration.

Keep asking for higher help and intervention in any area of your life. Then follow your intuition and lower your barriers. Let go of any notions of how Divinity will bring about your deepest heart's yearning. It may not be in the package you would expect but it will be life altering.

Your heart is about to be challenged to open wider than ever before. That may require you to feel some fear and pain. Do not run away from this experience. Take steps forward with faith that your greater good is coming.

ACTION

Place your hands on your heart. Ask yourself clearly what you desire. Imagine what it looks like and feels like to have this. Then surround this image with silver light. Imagine sending this image with the silver light into the middle of the universe. Ask that you receive this image or something much better.

Take a moment to reflect on feeling good like you already have the help you require.

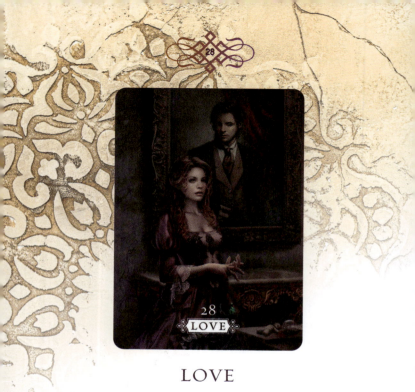

LOVE

Let go of your limiting beliefs about love.

Your heart desires more connections, love and nourishment. You are at a point in your life where you need to learn how to truly give and receive love.

Fully opening your heart will awaken your vulnerability, sensitivity and fear, in particular your fear of rejection and intimacy with another person. However, you will also unleash your passion, inspiration, greatness and an ability to care deeply.

Start seeing how great life is and be willing to connect to others. If you have been holding on to past pain then it is time to acknowledge, feel and move forward. Give yourself permission to let people in. Ask for love with all your heart and soul and it will come. Look for something beautiful in every person you encounter. Focus on feeling good, whenever you see people loving each other and know this is coming to you in a form of a love-of-a-lifetime or an incredible friendship.

ACTION

Focus on your heart. Take some slow, deep breaths. Imagine unlocking the door to your heart. What does your heart look like? Is it cold, frozen and dark? Or is it full of warmth, light and sweetness? If it is cold and grey, imagine melting the coldness with yellow light. Who do you need to communicate with so that your heart can heal? Imagine that this person is in front of you now. Say what you need to share without holding back. Now step into their shoes and answer back from the Highest Place within them.

Give yourself permission to experience an open heart. Every time you want to close your heart take some deep breaths and choose to keep it open, even if it hurts.

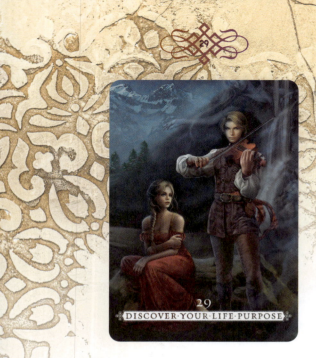

DISCOVER YOUR LIFE PURPOSE

Start asking yourself,
what is the meaning of your life?

As a soul who is having a physical experience you are here to grow and learn. You are being asked to immerse yourself in this life by expanding, stretching and understanding your reasons for being here.

Nothing is impossible for a soul who is following her or his destiny. Your guides, angels and Higher Self are constantly communicating with you through signs, feelings, people, books and so on.

Follow your hunches. You are being given important guidance, which may show up via a strong feeling to travel somewhere, to speak to someone, attend a seminar, write, paint and so on. No matter how far-fetched your inner guidance is you need to listen.

Your soul's purpose includes a combination of experiences that your mind doesn't understand but that your soul needs to process to learn and grow. Some of these experiences will be enjoyable and heightened. Others will be challenging and cause you to struggle, but through them you will know yourself. Give yourself permission to focus on what really makes your heart sing and put your intensity of emotion into attracting what you desire.

ACTION

Ask questions such as: 'Divine Intelligence, help me to understand what is occurring in my life and how it is serving my spirit. What is the next step for me? What is my mission here?'

When you are asking these questions you need to give yourself some time and space to receive the answers. The answers may come from a book you read, a person you encounter or your inner self. Keep a journal of your insights.

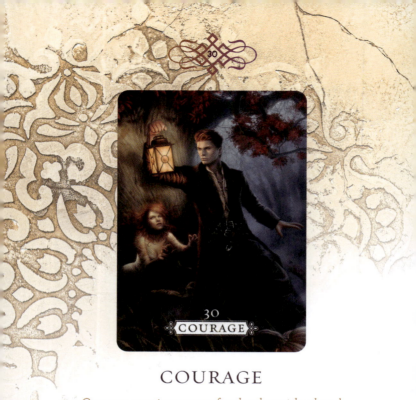

COURAGE

Courage requires you to fearlessly stride ahead despite the challenges you are experiencing.

Whether you are afraid of success or failure you cannot stay where you are. You need to make a decision and move forward with belief, trust and boldness. Give it your all, no matter the outcome.

Despite what you have been telling yourself, you are ready for a new adventure and another chance to prove that you have what it takes to face life's challenges. Stop investing in limitations, lack and dysfunction.

Every blessing has a challenge and every challenge contains a blessing. You are ready to explore both. Whilst there may be difficult moments ahead, keep positive and believe that everything is going to work out for your absolute best.

You are being asked to gather the courage to be who you truly are and to stand strong for your convictions.

ACTION

In order for you to succeed in what you desire you need to prepare for the challenges ahead.

Make a list of the support you need to tackle the approaching opportunities. Become aware of what or who you are afraid of. Imagine that this fear takes on the shape of a person. What does he or she look like? Look this fear in the eyes. Tell it that you are willing to learn from it and master the lesson, but you are not willing to be a slave to it. Imagine loving your fear and taking steps forward.

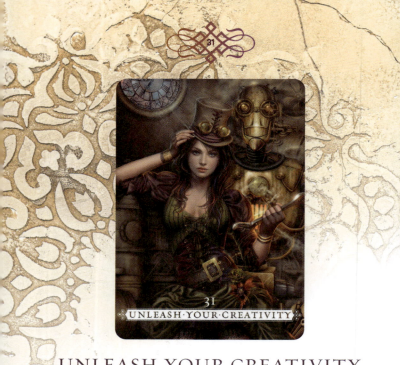

UNLEASH YOUR CREATIVITY

*Your creative talents and abilities are
your most powerful assets.*

Allow your imagination to roam without limits and access new ideas
without judging them.

It is time for you to be innovative and birth unique creations. If you are feeling stuck, get up and move, try new things, meet new people, read books, paint and so on.

Concentrate on the area of your life where you need to be creative. Are you a great singer who needs to share your talents with others? Do you have an affinity with gardening? Can you tell powerful stories? Are you technically minded? Can you whip up amazing meals? What is your special flavour of creativity?

Whatever it is, give yourself permission and the time to be inventive. The more creative you allow yourself to be, the more fulfilled you are going to feel.

ACTION

Focus on a challenge. Ask yourself, 'Is this true or are there other points of view I can adopt in relation to this issue?' Take some pencils and pens and draw these options, without judging or limiting them. Then stand up and ask your Higher Intelligence to show you new ways of doing things. Put on some music and dance. When the song ends, ask yourself, 'What other possibilities and creative ideas can I access?' Take a pen and paper and write them down.

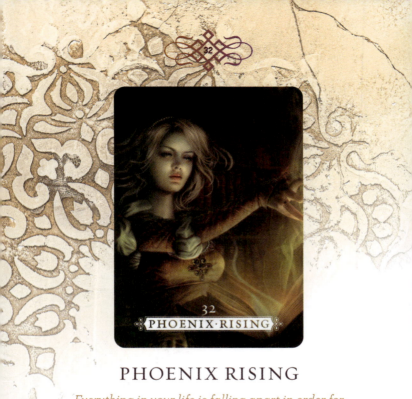

PHOENIX RISING

*Everything in your life is falling apart in order for
you to rise from the ashes with renewed strength.*

This is not a time to create but a time to sweep away everything that
has not worked in your life. The reason so many things are breaking

down and not going your way is because the old cycle of your life is completing.

You may feel that you are walking through the fires of life right now in order to be cleansed and purified for your rebirth. Soon you will not recognise yourself. You are reclaiming your spirit.

If possible, try to isolate yourself from the chaos surrounding you. Now is the time for you to feel any pain that you have previously suppressed so that you can heal. The universe has plans and opportunities that are better than you can imagine, so let go and trust and anticipate what is coming.

ACTION

Write down what you are afraid to let go of. Number your fears, from the worst thing that could happen to the smaller fears. Then write down what could be a possible gift of facing that fear.

Place your hands on the part of your body where you feel the most fear. Say to yourself or out loud, 'I am willing to let this fear go.' Imagine being able to take this sensation of fear out of your body and into the palms of your hands. Envisage that the fear becomes a bird. Surrender the bird to a Higher Source and visualise it flying away. Repeat the word 'surrender' several times.

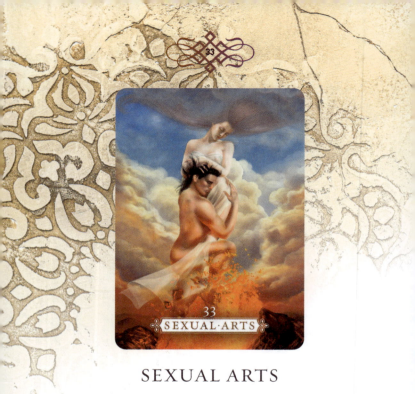

SEXUAL ARTS

Bring more light into your sexuality.

Keeping sexuality alive is an art form very few people truly understand.
Are you sexually attracted to your partner every day?
Sex energy only occurs where there is sexual polarity. Everyone has
both masculine and feminine qualities to gift each other. The only

time there is sexual spark is when one person is embodying more of their masculine energy and the other person is embodying more of their feminine energy.

The masculine is: the unchanging witness, presence, direction, decision-making, trying to bring everything to closure and consciousness itself.

The feminine is: change, life force, light, flowing movement, Mother Nature, emotions.

Do not buy into the myth that sexual attraction eventually dies in long-term relationships; sexual polarity is an art that takes practice; it can be so subtle and last a lifetime if you are constantly reinventing your gifts and using an open heart.

ACTION

Feminine essence people: instead of directly telling your masculine partner what you want, as this tends to kill polarity, invite him into action through expressing your feelings; your speech could be erotic and enticing instead of functional and efficient. Let him know how you're feeling and let him be inspired to direct you there.

Masculine essence people: your greatest gift is constant presence. No matter what your feminine partner is feeling or doing, constantly penetrate her display and see the light that is shining for you. The feminine may come at you like a slap to the face or your favourite kiss. Stay with her energy so the feminine knows that no matter what she's feeling you are there.

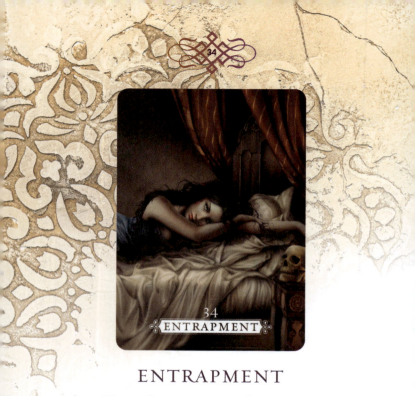

ENTRAPMENT

You are letting too many things in your environment control your life.

You have drawn this card because it is time for a shift in personal power. You are encouraged to take responsibility for your life and choose new ways of thinking that create change.

The reality is that for you to make the changes you want, need and desire, you need a system, daily discipline and motivation. As long as you blame outside influences for any circumstances in your life, you are powerless – it's the government, your abusive background, the interest rates, and the bank's fault.

The system that many ultra-successful people use is: they read books every day, listen to audios, go to as many seminars as they can, practise recognising other's achievements and form relationships with like-minded people.

ACTION

Ask yourself, 'Are the people in my life building me up and inspiring me?' If not, it is time to take charge and to start making change in your environment. Your first step could be cutting out all negative media from your daily life.

Another important action could involve changing your diet, cutting out sugar, food with MSG and GMO and replacing them with fresh, organic vegetables.

Take a moment and say the following statement to yourself or out aloud, 'I am in control of my life. Nothing can affect me unless I choose to let it. My thoughts create my reality.' Keep repeating this statement until you feel stronger. Eventually you will believe it. It will help you to make new choices. Remember, your words and self-talk are very powerful in altering your physiology.

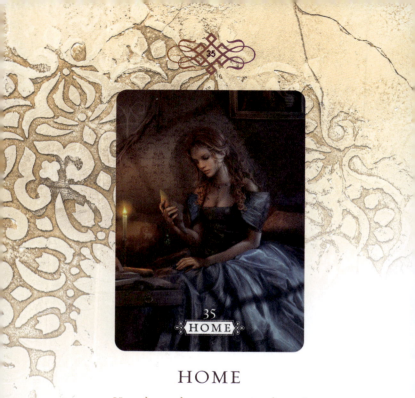

HOME

How do you keep re-creating home?

In the context of this teaching, let's use the word 'Home' to describe your unconscious ability to attract intimate partners with the positive and negative qualities your parents instilled in you.

This card honours the wounded child in you that keeps recreating Home, hoping to get your childhood developmental co-dependency needs met. You might even provoke the other to act or look like your original parent.

In a world where so many of our natural emotions were not encouraged and, worse yet, suppressed, you are now encouraged to feel the feelings trapped inside you and that consistently sabotage your life.

For some of us, Home was an amazing, empowering and happy place, but for most of us it was lacking; there was unease and hurt. This is imprinted on your nervous system, which forces the dysfunction you had with your parents to rise to the surface with your current partner and people close to you.

ACTION

Maybe your guardians' faces didn't show you love through the vital stages of development? Maybe there was abandonment or abuse?

Have courage, now, to feel where that frozen pain is stored and grieve. Use music, photos, movement and memories to connect with your inner child. Touch your body to intensify the sensations you are experiencing, with the intention of releasing stuck emotions.

An evolved partner or friend can roleplay with you by offering you a non-judgemental and kind gaze as you express your story or feelings. Then your partner can play the role of your parent and tell you that you are lovable. Spend time communicating with the little you and be gentle and loving.

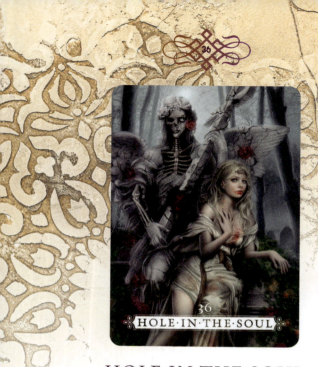

36

HOLE·IN·THE·SOUL

HOLE IN THE SOUL

*Your childhood wounds are
creating a hole in your soul.*

One way your childhood wounds disrupt an extraordinary life is
through low-grade depression experienced as a perpetual empty feeling.

If as a child you tried to make everything all right by picking up the pieces of your family dramas, then you adopted a false self. When you lose your authentic self you disconnect from your true feelings, needs and desires. Instead you wear a mask to make others feel more comfortable.

Being detached leads to profound loneliness and isolation as you are always mourning your true self.

This card encourages you to discover your true self through learning about your childhood and mourning the abandonment and neglect you felt.

ACTION

Find a safe place. Use coloured pencils to draw several masks. Each mask needs to represent an aspect of your false self such as a good girl/boy, saviour, slave, rebel, victim, overachiever and so on. Take time to write or draw the qualities you feel each false self contains.

Turn on some powerful music, put on a mask and move in a way you feel the mask requires for you to express yourself and feel the feelings you may have suppressed. Once you have completed the dance, take off the physical mask and burn it. Then imagine energetically taking off the false masks you wear in front of various people. Give yourself permission to be your real self. Imagine a person in front of you who you feel doesn't accept you. Say, 'I am going to betray you now and recover my true self.' Now imagine this person saying to you, 'I understand you and encourage you to become the person you were meant to be.'

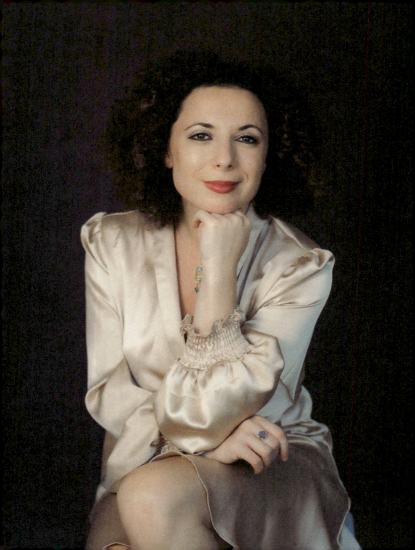

ABOUT THE AUTHOR

Inna is an internationally recognised healer, teacher, professional speaker, author and pioneer in the field of energy medicine and human consciousness. By intuitive means, she can 'see' illness and blocks in a person's body, explain what is occurring, and guide people through self-healing processes. However, her focus is not just to help a person heal physically but to also help them reconnect to their spiritual divine nature and understand deeper aspects of evolution.

When Inna was a teenager, she suffered from severe back pain, anxiety and a skin disorder. In an incredible twist of fate, while meditating, Inna was able to receive help from the divine source and unlock her ability to intuitively see into her body. By asking pertinent questions she was able to discover the root of her pain, release heavy energies and emotions and heal herself. This experience awakened her intuitive abilities to see what is happening in other people's bodies and inner lives.

She is able to teach her students how to understand the symbolic ways that their body and soul communicate through metaphors, images, feelings, memories, colours, sensations, thoughts and symbols.

Inna Segal is the award-winning bestselling author of *The Secret Language of Your Body: The Essential Guide to Health and Wellness*, *Understanding Modern Spirituality*, *Healing Heart Oracle* and *Mystical Healing Oracle*.

Inna has also created a variety of helpful healing audios and in-depth online programs. Her mission is to help people to awaken their inner life and step onto their true path of wellness, creativity, and to acknowledge their gifts and abilities that their spirit has brought to them.

Her books, cards and events (both live and online) are based on deep ancient wisdom, combined with a modern understanding of what we need right now to be our best selves, and the processes which allow us to grow and expand in a safe, profound and lasting manner.

Her passion is to help people understand the hidden mysteries of our existence – in particular, where we came from, where we are at the present moment, and where we are going in our future incarnations.

She deeply believes that we have to become more conscious of spiritual realities, which help us to understand the most progressive ways to live.

Find her at innasegal.com or on facebook.com/InnaSegalAuthor

ABOUT THE ILLUSTRATORS

Cris Ortega

Cris Ortega is a Spanish digital artist and writer. She completed her studies as an Advanced Technician in Illustration at the Art School of Valladolid, and worked several years as Art Director in the advertising agency Sm2. At the moment she works full time as a freelance artist.

At the end of 2005 she began to work as illustrator for Norma Editorial, publishing with them her first artbook with written stories, *Forgotten*, an artbook series with three volumes that has been translated into several languages. Another artbook, *Nocturna*, was published in 2011 by Imagica Ediciones.

Her works have been published as book covers, puzzles and posters, videogames, in well known artbooks like *Exotique* and *Spectrum*, in a lot of merchandising products and games and have been shown in several exhibitions.

To see more of Cris' work, visit www.crisortega.com

Drazenka Kimpel

Drazenka Kimpel is an awarded, licensed, digital illustrator who has worked on projects for a variety of gaming, comic and publishing companies around the world, as well as for corporate and private clients.

Her work has been featured in international publications such as *Expose, Exotique, D'artiste, Digital Art Masters, ImagineFX Magazine, Layers Magazine, Digital Arts Magazine* and many websites and online forums.

Drazenka is completely self-taught in design and illustration. Her style of painting is greatly influenced by the Neoclassical and Pre-Raphaelite masters, through their use of colour and narrative surroundings. She is highly fond of fantasy as a base for her subject matter, which gives her essential freedom to depict her own style of unknown visions, with romantic undertones and human interaction. Her ability to adapt to different styles of painting and design has helped her to work on different marketing campaigns.

To see more of Drazenka's work, visit creativedust.com

ACKNOWLEDGEMENTS

I profoundly thank my children Angelina and Raphael for your warmth, light, dedication and willingness to learn, grow and evolve. I am moved by your love, your depth and courage!

I also want to thank my family for all the support and challenges they have offered me so that I can keep learning, exploring and transforming.

My profound appreciation to Dianne Wynne for her absolute selfless dedication to helping people evolve. Thank you for all you do!

I thank all my students, readers and people who have touched my heart! There are too many of you to mention but you know who you are.

A special thank you to my most loyal and always supportive friend Piotr.

I'd like to thank Rudolf Steiner, Kevin Trudeau, David Deida and John Bradshaw from the depth of my heart for their outstanding contribution to humanity.

It is my hope that you will love the powerful images which the illustrators have contributed and that they will impact your soul as they have impacted mine. Thank you Cris and Drazenka, you are masters of your art.

To the Rockpool Publishing team, thank you for all your patience, enthusiasm and support! In particular my deep appreciation to Lisa and Paul for always being so understanding, encouraging and available.

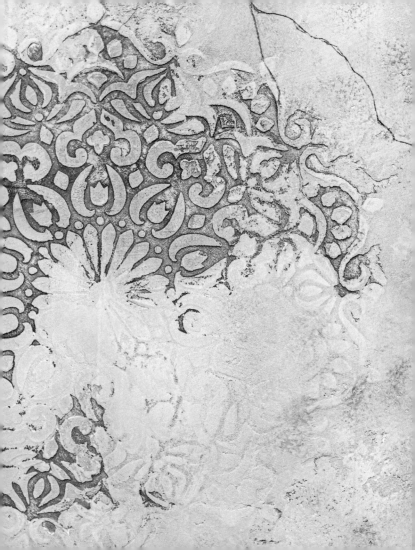